Current Hospital Medicine (CHM) is intended to be a quick reference guide for management of common medical conditions encountered in the inpatient hospital setting. It is envisioned to be a useful resource for medical students, interns, residents, advance practice providers and hospitalists.

CHM includes evidence based information with emphasis on initial treatment and management of patients who are being admitted to the hospital.

Medical students will find CHM useful during clinical rotations and while preparing for various clinical knowledge based exams. I believe this book will also be helpful to residents working under supervision during residency training. By referencing to CHM frequently, residents should be able to understand and follow recommendations from attending physicians easily and quickly, as is expected during busy medical floor rounds.

For hospitalist physicians and advanced practice providers, CHM can serve both as a quick reference and a refresher text. Hospitalists, nurse practitioners and physician assistants should use this book especially when admitting new patients to make sure all the standard care orders have been placed.

I hope that you find CHM useful throughout the continuous journey of learning medicine and taking care of our patients.

Amil Rafiq, MD

NOTICE

Medicine is an ever-changing science. As new research and clinical experience broaden our knowledge, changes in treatment and drug therapy are required. Although every effort has been made to make sure all the information is up to date, readers should still not rely solely on this book for making medical decisions. Medical information in this book is not intended as a substitute for professional care. Any recommendation in the book should be integrated with complete clinical picture.

Table of Contents

Section I

Acute Kidney Injury (AKI)/Acute Renal Failure 9
Alcohol Withdrawal _____ 11
Altered Mental Status (AMS) _____ 14
Anaphylactic Reaction/ Angioedema _____ 16
Asthma Exacerbation _____ 18
Atrial Fibrillation with RVR _____ 20
Bradycardia _____ 23
Candida UTI _____ 25
Cellulitis _____ 27
CHF Exacerbation _____ 29

CHM 5

Cholecystitis _____ *31*

Clostridioides (formerly Clostridium) Difficile Infection _____ *33*

COPD Exacerbation _____ *35*

Cyclical Vomiting Syndrome (Acute Flare Up) *37*

Deep Venous Thrombosis (DVT) _____ *39*

Diabetic Ketoacidosis (DKA) _____ *42*

Diverticulitis _____ *44*

GI Bleed _____ *46*

Helicobacter Pylori (HP) _____ *49*

Hepatic Encephalopathy _____ *51*

Heparin Induced Thrombocytopenia _____ *53*

Hypertriglyceridemia Induced Pancreatitis (HTGP) _____ *55*

Hyperkalemia _____ *57*

Hypertensive Emergency _____ *59*

Hypomagnesemia _____ *61*

Hyponatremia _____ *62*

Meningitis _____ *65*

6 CHM

Neutropenic Fever _____ 68

Non ST Elevation Acute Coronary Syndrome (NSTEACS) _____ 70

Orthostatic Hypotension _____ 73

Pancreatitis _____ 75

Pericarditis _____ 78

Pneumonia _____ 80

Pulmonary Embolism (PE) _____ 83

Pyelonephritis _____ 86

QTc Prolongation/ Acquired long QT syndrome (LQTS) _____ 88

Rhabdomyolysis _____ 89

Seizure _____ 90

Sepsis _____ 92

Sickle Cell Crisis (Acute Pain Episodes) _____ 94

Small Bowel Obstruction (SBO) _____ 97

Stroke/ Acute Cerebrovascular Accident (CVA) _____ 99

Supraventricular Tachycardia (SVT) _____ 103

Syncope _____ *105*
Tylenol Overdose _____ *107*

Section II

ABG Basics _____ *110*
Supplemental Oxygen _____ *114*
Noninvasive Ventilation _____ *117*
Mechanical Ventilation _____ *120*
EKG Basics _____ *123*
Supplement I: _____ *127*
Supplement II: _____ *130*
Supplement III: _____ *132*
Supplement IV: _____ *137*

Section I

Acute Kidney Injury (AKI)/Acute Renal Failure

- Send UA, Urine Electrolytes (Sodium, Creatinine)
- Give NS bolus 1 L followed by continuous infusion @125 mL/hr.

- Check FENa (< 1 pre-renal, > 2 ATN, value between 1 to 2 can be either pre-renal or ATN)

- Strict input and output monitoring
- Watch for fluid overload
- Order renal ultrasound

- Renal panel daily. Monitor potassium and phosphate levels

- Avoid nephrotoxic agents/ contrast. No NSAID's. No ACEI/ ARB's. No Diuretics.

- Avoid drastic lowering of blood pressure in order to maintain a good renal perfusion

- Monitor for potentially life-threatening complications of AKI including volume overload, refractory hyperkalemia, severe metabolic acidosis (pH <7.1), and any signs of uremia such as pericarditis, or an otherwise unexplained decline in mental status

- If serum phosphate concentrations is > 6 mg/dL, start on dietary phosphate binders like Sevelamer or Calcium acetate to be given with meals.

<u>In addition, in severe AKI</u> (increase in serum creatinine to 3 times baseline)

- Check pH, if <7.1 and patient not in fluid overload, start on Bicarb drip and consult nephrology.

<u>Hypervolemic patients</u>

- Patients with pulmonary edema/CHF, okay to use diuretic therapy in presence of AKI, typical initial dose of Lasix is 80 mg IV once.

Alcohol Withdrawal

- Give Banana bag x 1
- Check CBC, CMP, Mag, Phos, Serum alcohol level, Urine toxicology screen
- Start on continuous telemonitoring

- Should get CT head in patients with significant confusion or history of fall
- Lorazepam (Ativan) IV/PO as per CIWA protocol.
- Diazepam (Valium) 10 mg IV every 10 minutes x 3 doses can be used as initial therapy or symptom control in patients with severe withdrawal (avoid in patients with alcoholic hepatitis/cirrhosis).

- Start on IV fluids (D5NS @ 150 mL/hr)
- Strict input and output monitoring.
- Watch for fluid overload especially in cirrhotic patients.

- Use Chlordiazepoxide (Librium) 25 mg TID in patients able to take PO (Oxazepam 10 mg TID in patients with alcoholic hepatitis/cirrhosis). Taper and wean off Chlordiazepoxide prior to discharge

- Thiamine. Folic acid
- Give IV thiamine 100 mg daily initially, switch to PO in 48 to 72 hrs.

- Monitor electrolytes daily including Mag/Phos.

- Use Clonidine (usually as a patch) for treatment of uncontrolled hypertension in alcohol withdrawal

- Patients needing frequent/ high doses of sedatives, or worsening acidosis/ respiratory failure, transfer to ICU for close monitoring.

- Counsel patient about the health risks of alcohol and encourage quitting when patient stable and alcohol withdrawal resolved. Social worker referral for alcohol abuse rehab programs.

Alcohol withdrawal seizures

- No role for routine anticonvulsant therapy
- Can be managed with IV Lorazepam.

Alcoholic hepatitis

- Calculate DF (Maddrey discriminant function)

- Prednisolone 40 mg daily can be used in patients with DF ≥32, as 28-day course, followed by taper.

- If steroids are contraindicated, Pentoxifylline 400 mg TID can be used instead and continued until bilirubin falls below 5 mg/dL.

Altered Mental Status (AMS)

- Check CBG to rule out hypoglycemia
- Pulse oximetry, supplemental oxygen as needed (Target SpO2>88%)
- Send BMP, CBC, Mg, Ph, LFT's
- EKG and Cardiac enzymes
- ABG, CXR, UA

- Keep NPO until safe to swallow, start on gentle IV hydration (NS@ 75 mL/hr)
- Give IV thiamine (in alcoholics, malnourished, ESRD and cancer patients)

- TSH, B12, Folate, Cortisol, Ammonia level, Urine drug screen if indicated

- Blood cultures, Lactic acid, PCT if an infectious etiology is suspected.

- CT Head if persistent confusion, patient lethargic or unable to follow commands.

- MRI brain in selected cases with high suspicion of central causes

- Minimize narcotics and other drugs that could potentially cause worsening of mental status.

- Lumbar Puncture and EEG, if above work up is negative.

- Olanzapine/ Ativan PRN for severe agitation.

- Orientation protocols - provision of clocks, calendars, windows with outside views, frequent reassurance, touch, and verbal orientation especially from familiar persons.

Anaphylactic Reaction/ Angioedema

- Epinephrine 0.3 to 0.5 mg IM urgently in patients with lip swelling/ changes in voice. Can repeat dose every 5 to 15 minutes.

- Supplemental oxygen, 8 to 10 L/minute via facemask or 15 L/minute using a nonrebreather mask

- Start on IV fluids, NS @ 125 mL/hr.
- In hypotensive patients, treat aggressively with NS boluses

- Consider giving methylprednisolone 125 mg IV and continue on IV steroids, such as solumedrol 40 to 60 mg every 6 to 8 hours.

- Albuterol nebulization as needed for bronchospasm

- IV Pepcid BID. PRN Antihistaminics

- In patients with significant throat or tongue swelling, consider early intubation

- Cricothyroidotomy may be necessary if attempts at intubation fail.

- Prescribe EpiPen and refer to allergist/immunologist, upon discharge

Asthma Exacerbation

- Supplemental O2 as needed to target a SpO2 of > 92% (> 95% in pregnant patients)

- Bronchodilators – Albuterol 2.5 mg nebulization every 20 minutes for three doses, then 2.5 mg every 4 to 6 hours as needed.

- CXR, if indicated (patients with significant cough/sputum production).

- For patients with severe exacerbations, add Ipratropium 0.5 mg by nebulization every 20 minutes for 3 doses (DuoNeb- albuterol plus ipratropium) plus one dose of Magnesium sulfate 2 grams IV over 20 minutes.

- Check for COVID and influenza/ viral panel during the fall and winter seasons.

- Start on PO steroids, Prednisone 40 to 60 mg daily. Consider IV Steroids (Solumedrol

60 to 80 mg every 8 to 12 hours) only in very severe exacerbations/ ICU patients.

- Consult pulmonology for severe/ recurrent exacerbations.

- Titrate steroids as per clinical response. Continue prednisone 40 mg daily upon discharge for 5 days and provide prescription for inhaled glucocorticoid (such as Flovent HFA, low dose 110 mcg twice daily)

Atrial Fibrillation with RVR

- Give Metoprolol 5 mg IV q 5 mins (total 15 mg) or Diltiazem 20 mg IV (can repeat dose in 15 min's)

- If rate control is achieved, start on scheduled PO Metoprolol or Diltiazem

- If rate control is not achieved with IV bolus medications, start on Diltiazem or Esmolol drip (without extra drip bolus)

- Check BMP, Mg and TSH levels.
- Supplement electrolytes, Keep K > 4, Mg > 2
- Start on continuous telemonitoring and order ECHO.

- Closely monitor blood pressure while on IV drip medications. Hold if systolic blood pressure drops < 90

- Once heart rate is maintained less than 100, begin oral Diltiazem regimen

- Oral Diltiazem is typically started at 30 mg every 6 hours or 60 mg every 8 hours. Taper and discontinue infusion 2 hours after second oral dose.

- For conversion from Esmolol drip, stop the drip and start on PO Metoprolol 25 mg BID (or 12.5 mg BID, if BP on lower side)

- Oral medications should be changed to sustained release formulations prior to discharge

- Patients who do not respond to or are intolerant of IV Metoprolol/ Cardizem; start on Amiodarone drip and consult cardiology.

- Evaluate all patients for benefits of oral anticoagulation (CHADS2-Vasc score) vs risk of bleeding (HAS- BLED score, recurrent falls)

Patients with advanced HF or borderline hypotension

- Digoxin 0.5 mg IV once, can be used as initial therapy, typically begins to act in 15 to 30 minutes.

- Repeat doses of 0.25 mg every 6 hours to a maximum loading dose of 1.5 mg over 24 hours (0.75 mg in renal failure patients).

- Maintenance dose between 0.125 mg and 0.25 mg daily based on weight/renal function

Bradycardia

- Start on continuous tele monitoring, pulse oximetry and get 12 lead EKG

- Stop any offending drugs such as beta blockers, calcium channel blockers and digoxin

- Check trop's, TSH, electrolytes (BMP, Mg, Phos)

- For asymptomatic patients continue observation

- For symptomatic patients (lightheadedness, chest pain, sob, confusion, presyncope or syncope), and patients with hemodynamic instability (hypotension) give Atropine 1 mg IV push, repeat every 3 to 5 mins for a total dose of 3 mg.

- If Atropine ineffective, can start on Dopamine IV infusion 5 mcg/kg per min and titrate up to 20 mcg/kg per min **OR** Epinephrine IV infusion 2 to 10 mcg per min.

- Transcutaneous pacing and cardiology consult for possible transvenous pacing or permanent pacemaker placement.

Candida UTI

- Majority of fungal UTI's are caused by Candida albicans

- Once UA shows yeast, culture that specimen and send another culture to rule out contamination

- Asymptomatic candiduria is common in hospitalized patients and does not require treatment except in neutropenic patients and those undergoing urological procedure.

- Indwelling catheters should be removed or replaced when possible.

- If patient is symptomatic, start on Fluconazole 200 mg daily for 14 days

- If pyelonephritis is suspected, give Fluconazole 400 mg daily for 14 days

- For fluconazole resistant Candida such as C. Glabrata, switch to Amphotericin B after consultation with ID.

- Neutropenic patients with candiduria: Consult ID as these patients are presumed to have disseminated infection (Typical antifungal regimen: Micafungin 100 mg IV daily)

Cellulitis

- Check PCT, LA, ESR, CRP.
- Send blood cultures.

- Elevate the affected area/limb
- If septic, begin aggressive hydration

- Start on IV antibiotics
    - Vancomycin and Zosyn (Severe infection)
    - Ceftriaxone **OR** Unasyn **OR** Ciprofloxacin plus Clindamycin (Mild to moderate infection)

- Send wound culture if any open wounds/purulent discharge.

- In patients with significant swelling/edema get venous duplex to rule out DVT, and consider CT with contrast to rule out abscess or deep infection (especially in patients with hyponatremia, elevated CPK or AST)

- In patients with ulcers or cellulitis of toes, get X-rays to rule out osteomyelitis (OM). Might need MRI if clinical suspicion high and X-ray negative for OM

- Duration of therapy is individualized depending on clinical response, typically ranges between 5 to 14 days.

CHF Exacerbation

- Supplemental O2 as needed, goal SpO2 > 90%. ABG, BiPAP- If significant hypoxia present

- Elevate head end of bed 30 to 45 degrees
- Continuous telemonitoring

- Start on IV Lasix 40 to 80 mg daily (in divided doses). Patients on chronic diuretics, typical IV doses are usually 2 to 2.5 times the daily oral dose.

- Strict input and output monitoring.
- Fluid restriction and daily weights

- EKG, Serial trop's, CXR, ECHO
- Check BNP, repeat in 48 hrs.
- Monitor renal function and electrolytes. Keep K > 4, Mg > 2

- Patients with known aortic stenosis – use diuretics with caution

Approach to refractory heart failure and hypotension

- Start on Dobutamine, run continuously at 2.5 mcg/kg per min to help in diuresis. Can uptitrate to 10 mcg/kg per min to maintain MAP> 65.

Long term management of patients with HFrEF

- Start on low dose ACE inhibitor (such as Enalapril 2.5 mg) and Beta blocker (such as Carvedilol 3.125 mg BID) prior to discharge.

- Entresto (Sacubitril-valsartan) is now preferred over ACE inhibitor for patients with LVEF ≤40 % provided there are no cost constraints, might need insurance approval.

- Consider starting on Sodium-glucose cotransporter 2 (SGLT2) inhibitors such as Jardiance (Empagliflozin) 10 mg daily in all patients with or without type 2 diabetes.

- Consider IV Iron supplementation in patients with Ferritin <100 ng/mL.

Cholecystitis

- Keep NPO except med's and start on IV hydration. Monitor electrolytes.

- Supportive care with pain control (Toradol, Morphine) and antiemetics as needed

- If diagnosis is inconclusive on initial imaging (USG/CT) get HIDA scan

- Send CBC, CMP, PCT, LA and Blood cultures

- Start on IV antibiotics such as Zosyn 3.375 g IV every 6 hours **OR** Ceftriaxone 2 g IV once daily **OR** Levofloxacin 750 mg IV or PO once daily

- Subsequently, can start on clears and advance diet as tolerated

- Consult surgery team for definitive therapy (cholecystectomy) during same hospitalization.

- Continue antibiotics until gallbladder is removed or cholecystitis resolved.

- If symptoms do not improve with supportive care and risk of cholecystectomy outweighs the potential benefits, then gallbladder drainage (percutaneous cholecystostomy) is indicated

Approach to dilated CBD

- Patients with acute cholangitis (fever/chills or leukocytosis; with bilirubin ≥ 2 or abnormal LFT's; and biliary dilation on imaging) or with evidence of stone in CBD proceed directly with ERCP. Other patients can consider MRCP first.

Clostridioides (formerly Clostridium) Difficile Infection

- Contact precautions, hand hygiene with soap and water

- Start on Fidaxomicin 200 mg orally twice daily for 10 days (Drug of choice) **OR** Vancomycin 125 mg orally 4 times daily x 10 days (Preferred if cost constraints)

- Supportive care with IV fluids, correction of electrolyte imbalances
- Clear liquid diet, advance as tolerated.

- For patients with fulminant colitis (hypotension, ileus, megacolon) get CT abdomen/ pelvis, start on PO Vancomycin (500 mg four times daily) plus IV Metronidazole (500 mg every 8 hours), consult ID and consider early surgical consultation.

- If unable to take PO, can give Vancomycin via nasogastric tube or as retention enema (if Ileus present)

- For first recurrence can repeat Fidaxomicin 200 mg orally twice daily for 10 days **OR** Vancomycin 125 mg orally 4 times daily for 10 days

- For second recurrence can again repeat Fidaxomicin 200 mg orally twice daily for 10 days **OR** use Vancomycin pulsed-tapered regimen (Vancomycin 125 mg orally 4 times daily for 14 days, then 125 mg orally twice daily for 7 days, then 125 mg orally once daily for 7 days, then 125 mg orally every other day for 2 weeks)

- For patients with multiple recurrences consider fecal microbiota transplantation (FMT)

COPD Exacerbation

- Supplemental O2 as needed to target SpO2 of 88 to 92 percent. ABG, BiPAP as needed.

- Albuterol 2.5 mg and Ipratropium 0.5 mg nebulization (DuoNeb) every hour for three doses, then every 2 to 4 hours as needed.

- CXR to rule out concurrent pneumonia
- Sputum culture if possible.

- Check for COVID and influenza/ viral panel during the fall and winter seasons.

- Start on PO steroids, Prednisone 40 to 60 mg daily. Consider IV Steroids (Solumedrol 60 to 80 mg every 8 to 12 hours) only in very severe exacerbations/ ICU patients.

- Empiric antibiotics: Levofloxacin 500 mg PO/ IV **OR** Ceftriaxone 1 to 2 grams IV. Other oral options for milder exacerbations include Azithromycin **OR** Augmentin. Duration is typically 3 to 5 days.

- Consult pulmonology for severe/ recurrent exacerbations.

- If patient is started on BiPAP, repeat ABG in 2 hours. Consult ICU if repeat ABG worsened or pH <7.25 for possible intubation/ mechanical ventilation.

- Titrate steroids as per clinical response. Continue prednisone 40 mg daily upon discharge for 5 days.

Cyclical Vomiting Syndrome (Acute Flare Up)

- Start on IV fluids, D5NS @ 100 to 125 mL/hr

- Monitor electrolytes especially potassium, supplement as indicated

- Antiemetics (Zofran/ Reglan) as needed
- Zofran is antiemetic of choice with maximum total dose of 32 mg/24 hours

- Daily EKG to monitor QT interval

- Sedatives (Diphenhydramine/ Lorazepam) as needed to supplement antiemetics.

- Pain management- Tylenol, Toradol
- Minimize narcotic use
- Check urine toxicology for cannabinoids

- Trial of clears, advance diet as tolerated

Outpatient management

- Encourage patients to follow up with PCP to discuss abortive agents (such as Sumatriptan) and prophylactic therapy (such as Amitryptyline) in patients with frequent exacerbations.

Deep Venous Thrombosis (DVT)

- Start on IV UFH (Unfractionated Heparin) or SubQ LMWH (Lovenox)

- Typical dosing for UFH is 80 units/kg bolus (maximum dose: 10,000 units), then 18 units/kg/hour (maximum initial infusion: 2,000 units/hour). Dosing adjustment/ monitoring should be guided per pharmacy protocol/ local hospital heparin dosing nomogram

- Typical dosing for LMWH is 1 mg/kg every 12 hours or 1.5 mg/kg once daily. Avoid use or adjust dose to 1 mg/kg once daily in patients with CrCl <30 mL/minute

- Start on oral anticoagulation (OAC), usually after 24 hrs.

- For patients in whom anticoagulation is contraindicated consider IVC filter placement

- In patients with significant hypoxia/ SOB, get ABG and CT angio chest to rule out PE. If unable to get CT angio (due to renal failure, contrast allergy) get V/Q scan. If imaging positive for PE, start on continuous telemonitoring and get ECHO to check RVSP

- For patients with extensive iliofemoral DVT, consult interventional radiology/ vascular surgery for catheter-directed thrombolytic therapy/ surgical thrombectomy.

- LMWH is preferred in pregnancy, patients with history of cancer or liver disease with acquired coagulopathy

Transitioning from IV/SubQ to oral anticoagulation:

- Warfarin: Overlap IV Heparin or SubQ Lovenox with Warfarin until INR is therapeutic x 2

- Eliquis/Xarelto: Start direct-acting oral anticoagulant (DOAC) when heparin infusion is stopped or within 2 hours prior to the next scheduled dose of Lovenox

- DOAC Dosage:
    - Eliquis (Apixaban) 10 mg twice daily for 7 days followed by 5 mg twice daily.
    - Xarelto (Rivaroxaban) 15 mg twice daily with food for 21 days followed by 20 mg once daily with food.

- Warfarin is typically started at 5 mg once daily

Duration of therapy

- Provoked DVT/PE: Minimum 3 months
- First unprovoked DVT/PE: 3 months (if significant bleeding risk or patient refuses lifelong anticoagulation) to indefinite treatment (if low bleeding risk and patient agrees)
- First DVT/PE with active cancer: Indefinite treatment
- Second unprovoked DVT/PE: Indefinite treatment

Diabetic Ketoacidosis (DKA)

- CBC, BMP, ABG, urine ketones by dipstick, serum ketones (beta-hydroxybutyric acid)

- Start on aggressive IV hydration, NS bolus 1000 mL/hr for 2 to 3 hours and then continue NS @ 250 mL/hr
- Strict input and output monitoring

- Insulin drip as per DKA protocol
- Check BMP every 4 hours.
- Supplement Potassium as needed, goal K > 4, If Potassium falls < 3.3, hold Insulin drip and replace potassium first.
- Consider Bicarb replacement only if arterial pH ≤ 6.9

- Monitor glucose levels, CBG checks every 1 to 2 hours.
- If anion gap is still elevated and CBG falls < 200 mg/dL, change IV fluids to D5 1/2 NS @ 150 to 250 mL/hr.

- Once anion gap is closed (<18), start on diet and initiate home (pre-DKA) subcutaneous Insulin regimen. In Insulin-naive patients, start long acting insulin (Levemir/ Lantus) at a dose of 0.5 units/kg per day, plus sliding scale insulin.
- Continue IV Insulin drip for atleast 2 hours after giving subcutaneous Insulin

- Monitor blood sugars AC/HS and adjust subcutaneous Insulin regimen as needed.
- Consult dietician/ diabetes education nurse

Of note:
- Treatment of hyperosmolar hyperglycemic state (HHS) is similar to that of DKA.

- Subcutaneous insulin protocols (instead of Insulin drip) can be used in selected patients with mild to moderate DKA

- Reactive leukocytosis unrelated to infection and elevated serum amylase/ lipase levels without acute pancreatitis can be seen in patients with DKA

Diverticulitis

- Keep NPO except med's and start on IV hydration. Monitor electrolytes.

- Supportive care with pain control (Toradol, Morphine) and antiemetics as needed

- Send CBC, BMP, PCT, LA and Blood cultures

- Start on IV antibiotics such as Zosyn 3.375 g IV every 6 hours **OR** Ceftriaxone 2 g IV once daily plus Metronidazole 500 mg IV or PO every 8 hours **OR** Levofloxacin 750 mg IV or PO once daily plus Metronidazole 500 mg IV or PO every 8 hours

- Trials of clears in 24 to 48 hrs, advance diet as tolerated

- Once tolerating diet, can switch antibiotics to PO (Augmentin **OR** Levaquin plus Flagyl) to complete a total of 10 to 14 days course.

- If patient fails to improve within 48 to 72 hrs or shows any signs of worsening, get CT abdomen pelvis with contrast to rule out abscess or perforation.

Approach to complications of acute diverticulitis

- In patients with microperforation (contained perforation), continue conservative management with IV antibiotics.
- Patients with frank perforation (free air under the diaphragm), emergent surgery is indicated.
- Patients with abscess < 4 cm, can continue conservative management with IV antibiotics and serial CT scans until the resolution. Any abscess ≥4 cm, should undergo CT guided drainage. If abscess is not amenable to percutaneous drainage, can continue with IV antibiotics and monitor closely with serial CT scans. If no improvement in 2 to 3 days, surgery is indicated.

GI Bleed

- CBC, BMP, LFT, PT/INR
- Keep NPO and start on maintenance IV fluids NS @ 75 mL/hr
- Continuous telemonitoring

- Start on PPI (proton pump Inhibitor): Pantoprazole 80 mg IV once and then continue 40 mg IV BID

- Monitor hemoglobin/hematocrit closely (every 6 to 12 hours depending on severity of bleed)

- For majority of patients, transfuse PRBCs as needed for Hb < 8 g/dL. In patients with cirrhosis, Hb > 7 g/dL is acceptable. For patients with active bleeding or hemodynamic instability or acute MI can transfuse for Hb < 10 g/dL.

- Give FFP (fresh frozen plasma) for coagulopathy (elevated INR)

- Give platelets for thrombocytopenia (platelets <50,000) or platelet dysfunction in patients on chronic aspirin therapy.

- Patients who receive multiple units of PRBCs should also get FFP and platelets (typically after transfusing four units of PRBCs)

- Avoid any NSAID's or Aspirin

- Consult Gastroenterology for EGD+/- Colonoscopy

In addition, in variceal bleed

- Give Octreotide 50 mcg bolus, followed by 50 mcg/hour infusion to be continued for 3 to 5 days.

Patients with cirrhosis

- Start on prophylactic antibiotic such as Ceftriaxone 1 g IV daily, can change to Ciprofloxacin 500 mg PO BID upon discharge to complete a total of 7 days of antibiotic therapy.

Patients on oral anticoagulants

- Warfarin: Vitamin K 10 mg IV and FFP 2 units or PCC (prothrombin complex concentrate/ Kcentra). INR check 15 minutes after infusion is complete. If INR still > 1.5 can give additional FFP 2 units or PCC.

- DOACs (Xarelto/Eliquis): PCC (Kcentra) and tranexamic acid

Helicobacter Pylori (HP)

- Check HP IgG. No further work-up if HP IgG negative.
- If H pylori serology positive, confirm HP infection with HP stool or HP breath test outpatient (Patient needs to be off PPI for atleast a week)

- If stool or breath test positive, treat with two antibiotics and PPI for 10-14 days.

- Commonly used regimen: Omeprazole 20 mg twice a day, amoxicillin 1 g twice a day, clarithromycin 500 mg twice a day (OAC) for 10 days.

- Confirm eradication with stool or breath test after another 6 weeks (again off PPI x 1 week pre-test)

- Serum qualitative antibody test remains positive after treatment.

- Stool antigen test is useful to detect active infections or monitor response to therapy.

Hepatic Encephalopathy

- CBC, CMP, PT/INR, UA, CXR, Blood cultures, Ammonia and Alcohol level

- Noncontrast CT head in patients with coagulopathy, significant mental status changes or history of fall (may show cerebral edema)

- Lactulose 20 gram every 4 hrs initially. Titrate to achieve 2 to 3 soft stools per day. If patient unable to take PO, can use Lactulose enemas.

- If no adequate response within 24 to 48 hrs, add Rifaximin 400 mg TID or 550 mg BID.

- Monitor electrolytes, supplement as indicated
- Consider gentle hydration, avoiding dehydration.

- Evaluate and treat any precipitating factors like infection, sedatives, dehydration, GI bleed, constipation, electrolyte abnormalities, portal or hepatic vein thrombosis.

- Use of restraints for agitation, may be a safer option than pharmacologic treatment. Should medications be required, Haloperidol is a safer option than benzodiazepines.

Approach to patients with ascites

- Abdominal ultrasound and paracentesis are recommended to rule out spontaneous bacterial peritonitis (SBP).
- Elevated INR or thrombocytopenia is not a contraindication to paracentesis
- In patients with abdominal pain and unremarkable routine workup, consider Doppler ultrasonography/ contrast enhanced CT of abdomen to rule out portal vein thrombosis or hepatic vein thrombosis (Budd-Chiari syndrome).

Of note: If Rifaximin is initiated, continue for atleast 3 months.

Heparin Induced Thrombocytopenia

- Patients with HIT are at high risk for both venous and arterial thrombosis

- Discontinue all Heparins, and Warfarin (in patients chronically on Warfarin)
- Send HIT (PF4) antibody

- If clinical suspicion is high (4 Ts score: 4 to 8 points), start on non-heparin anticoagulant while awaiting definitive test results in consultation with Hem/Onc

- Direct oral anticoagulants (DOACs) Apixaban (Eliquis) or Rivaroxaban (Xarelto) can be used as initial non-heparin anticoagulant

- Patients with acute thrombosis, planned invasive procedure or higher risk of bleeding, use Argatroban drip **OR** Fondaparinux (dosing per pharmacy).

- Check venous duplex of bilateral lower extremities to rule out DVT

- **Transitioning to Warfarin:**
  - Start on low dose (5 mg) warfarin when platelet count >150K.
  - Need a minimum of five days of overlapping therapy
  - When INR is > 4 on combined warfarin and argatroban therapy
    - Stop Argatroban drip
    - Repeat INR measurement in 4 to 6 hours
    - If INR is below therapeutic level, resume argatroban therapy
    - Repeat procedure daily until desired INR on warfarin alone is obtained

- **Duration of treatment:**
  - HIT without thrombosis: treat for 4 weeks
  - HIT with thrombosis: treat atleast for 3 months

Hypertriglyceridemia Induced Pancreatitis (HTGP)

- Hypertriglyceridemia is suspected as etiology of acute pancreatitis in patients with serum triglyceride levels atleast > 500 mg/dL (5.6 mmol/L) typically >1000 mg/dL (11.2 mmol/L)

- Keep NPO and start on aggressive IV hydration (NS@150 mL/hr)
- Strict input and output monitoring
- Monitor serum electrolytes (ionized Ca /Mg), supplement as indicated.
- Supportive care with pain control (Morphine, Fentanyl) and antiemetics as needed

- Start on Insulin drip (0.1 to 0.3 units/kg/hour), monitor CBG's every hour and triglyceride levels/BMP every 12 hours.
- If CBG falls < 200 mg/dL, change IV fluids to D5 (Dextrose 5%)

- If Potassium falls < 3.3 mEq/L, then hold Insulin and replace potassium first.
- Discontinue insulin drip when triglyceride levels are < 500 mg/dL (5.6 mmol/L)

- Start on trial of clears when appropriate and advance to low fat diet as tolerated

- Start Gemfibrozil (600 mg BID) when tolerating diet

<u>Approach to multi drug therapy for hypertriglyceridemia</u>

- For patients who are already on a statin, consider adding icosapent ethyl (fish oil) 4 g daily. For patients who require combined therapy with a Statin and Fibrate, Fenofibrate (Fenofibric acid 145 mg daily) is preferred over Gemfibrozil due to lesser risk of muscle toxicity.

Hyperkalemia

- Pseudohyperkalemia due to hemolysis of the blood specimen is not uncommon and must be excluded first.

- Patients with muscle weakness, ECG changes or potassium > 6.5 mEq/L, start immediately on continuous telemonitoring and give Calcium gluconate 1 ampule (1000 mg) to stabilize cardiac membranes

  - Give IV bolus of regular insulin 10 units, followed immediately with 50 mL of a 50% Dextrose solution and check CBGs hourly for up to six hours to monitor for hypoglycemia.

  - Give Sodium zirconium cyclosilicate (SZC/ Lokelma) 10 g TID for 48 hours or Patiromer (Veltassa) 8.4 g daily as needed

  - Repeat BMP to check serum potassium levels in 2 hours. If potassium is still high, can repeat Insulin/Dextrose. Can also give furosemide 20 to 40 mg IV and/or albuterol nebulization.

- Hemodialysis, if conservative measures fail.

- In patients with mild to moderate hyperkalemia (potassium 5.5 – 6.5 mEq/L) Calcium gluconate is usually not indicated. Insulin/Dextrose is used on a case-by-case basis. Potassium can be reduced gradually with SZC, diuretics and a low-potassium diet.

- Discontinue medications that can contribute to hyperkalemia such as ACE inhibitors, ARBs, aldosterone antagonists, NSAIDs and nonselective beta blockers

Hypertensive Emergency

- Severe symptomatic hypertension (SBP >180 and/or DBP >120) with agitation, altered mental status, seizures, chest pain, shortness of breath or nausea/vomiting, requires emergent treatment.

- Start on continuous telemonitoring and IV antihypertensive medications such as Labetalol (0.5 to 2 mg/minute) or Nicardipine (5 to 15 mg/hour) drip.

- Serial troponins in patients with chest pain. Monitor renal function closely. If recurrent vomiting develops and/or any acute change in mental status get stat CT head

- Labetalol drip is acceptable in most patients except those with bradycardia, asthma/COPD, pheochromocytoma or cocaine/ methamphetamine overdose.

- Nicardipine drip is preferred if bradycardia present.

- Nitroglycerin drip (5 to 100 mcg/minute) is preferred in patients with acute pulmonary edema.

- Avoid drastic lowering of blood pressure, goal is to lower BP not more than 25 to 30 % in the first 24 hours.

- Once blood pressure is better controlled, wean off IV medications and switch to oral anti hypertensive medications

- In patients with severe but asymptomatic hypertension (hypertensive urgency) blood pressure reduction is considered non emergent, can trial oral agents such as Clonidine.

Hypomagnesemia

- IV supplementation:
    - Mg <1 mg/dL: give 4 grams of Magnesium sulphate.
    - Mg 1 to 1.5 mg/dL: give 2 grams of Magnesium sulphate
    - Mg 1.6 to 1.9 mg/dL: give 1 gram of Magnesium sulphate

- Oral supplementation:
    - Works better then IV supplementation (50% of IV magnesium is excreted back into urine) but has more GI side effects
    - Sustained-release preparation Magnesium chloride (SlowMag) 71.5 mg daily is better tolerated compared to Magnesium oxide (Mag-Ox) 400 mg BID

Hyponatremia

- Hyponatremia in patients that develops at home/outside hospital is usually categorized as chronic hyponatremia (been present for more than 48 hours, or duration unclear)

- Start on IV fluids, normal saline @ 100 mL/hr

- Send serum osmolality, TSH, lipid panel, urine sodium and urine osmolality

- Repeat BMP every 4 hours.

- Goal is to increase serum sodium initially by not more than 4 to 6 mEq/L during the first 24 hours (to prevent the risk of osmotic demyelination syndrome)

- In patients with severe hyponatremia (<120 mEq/L) or moderate hyponatremia (120 to 129 mEq/L) with severe symptoms such as seizures, obtundation, coma, or respiratory arrest, start on hypertonic 3% saline immediately at a rate of 15 to 30 mL/hour and consult nephrology urgently. Hypertonic saline can be administered via peripheral vein safely, placement of a central venous catheter is not necessary. Monitor serum sodium hourly while on hypertonic saline. If sodium is correcting too fast, stop hypertonic saline and start on D5W infusion.

- Patients with acute hyponatremia that has developed over a period of less than 48 hours even with mild symptoms should be considered for hypertonic saline after discussion with nephrology.

- In hypervolemic patients, restrict fluids and consider diuretics

- In patients with SIADH, sodium typically worsens with saline, start on fluid restriction (800 mL/day), might need salt tablets and diuretics.

SIADH clues
- A low serum osmolality
- An inappropriately elevated urine osmolality (> 100, usually > 300 mosmol/kg)
- A urine sodium concentration usually above 40 meq/L
- Low blood urea nitrogen and serum uric acid concentration
- A relatively normal serum creatinine concentration
- Normal acid-base and potassium balance
- Normal adrenal and thyroid function

Meningitis

- Suspect bacterial meningitis in patients with fever, headaches, altered mental status, and nuchal rigidity

- Initiate droplet precautions and collect two sets of blood cultures

- Get urgent lumbar puncture, give Dexamethasone (0.15 mg/kg) and start immediately on Ceftriaxone (2 gram IV every 12 hrs), Vancomycin (15 to 20 mg/kg IV every 8 to 12 hours as per pharmacy protocol), and Acyclovir (10 mg/kg of ideal body weight IV every 8 hrs)

- If age > 50 years, add ampicillin (2 gram every 4 hrs) to cover against *Listeria monocytogenes*

- Continue with dexamethasone (0.15 mg/kg every 6 hrs) only if *Streptococcus pneumoniae* is suspected on CSF Gram stain/cultures

- CT head is indicated prior to lumbar puncture in patients with altered mental status, focal neurologic deficit, new onset seizure, papilledema, history of CNS disease or immunocompromised state. Such patients can be started on empiric therapy immediately after collecting blood cultures.

- In patients with CSF shunt, recent history of neurosurgery, or penetrating head trauma, Ceftriaxone should be replaced with Cefepime (2 g IV every 8 hrs)

- Frequent neurochecks and continuous telemonitoring

- Check lactic acid, PCT and consider gentle IV hydration

- Consult ID and modify treatment based on CSF analysis and culture results.

Typical CSF findings:

- Bacterial meningitis: WBC > 1000, Glucose < 40, Protein > 100
- Viral meningitis: WBC < 500 (predominantly lymphocytes > 50%), normal Glucose, Protein < 100, negative Gram stain

Neutropenic Fever

- Supplemental O2 as needed to maintain SpO2 >90%

- Initiate neutropenic precautions in patients with severe neutropenia (ANC <500 cells/microL)

- Collect two sets of blood cultures and start on empiric IV antibiotics such as Cefepime 2 g IV every 8 hours, as soon as possible.

- Start on IV fluids, monitor urine output and serum electrolytes.

- Check Lactic acid, PCT, CXR, UA
- Influenza screen/ viral panel during the fall and winter seasons.
- Consider CT chest/abdomen/pelvis if UA/CXR negative

- In patients with sepsis, pneumonia, skin/soft tissue infection, or suspected central venous catheter (CVC) related infections, continue

Cefepime and add Vancomycin 15 to 20 mg/kg IV every 8 to 12 hours as per pharmacy protocol.

- Early ID consult recommended to modify antibiotic regimen as needed
- Hem/onc consultant should guide RBC and PLT transfusions

- Serial blood cultures in patients with bacteremia
- If symptoms warrant check stool for C Diff
- Consider CT sinuses and removal of any central venous catheters, if source of infection remains unclear.

- Patients who continue to be febrile with no apparent source of infection despite being on broad spectrum antibiotics for few days, consider addition of empiric antifungal agents after discussion with ID consultant.

Non ST Elevation Acute Coronary Syndrome (NSTEACS)

- Includes unstable angina and non-ST elevation myocardial infarction (NSTEMI)

- Start on continuous telemonitoring and supplemental O2 as needed to maintain SpO2 >90%

- Give Aspirin 162 to 325 mg to be chewed and swallowed. If unable to take PO give as rectal suppository

- Obtain serial EKG's and trend troponins (every 4 to 6 hrs)

- Give sublingual Nitroglycerin tablets (0.4 mg) every five minutes for maximum of three doses except in patients with hypotension or those using phosphodiesterase inhibitors. In patients with persistent symptoms, start on Nitroglycerin drip at 10 mcg/min and increase the drip rate by 10 mcg/min every 5 minutes until pain resolves or systolic BP falls below 100 mmHg

- Clopidogrel loading dose of 300 mg once, and then continue with 75 mg daily

- Give IV Heparin (UFH) bolus of 60 units/kg (maximum of 4000 units), followed by a continuous IV infusion of 12 units/kg/hour (maximum 1000 units/hour) adjusted per pharmacy protocol to achieve a goal aPTT of approximately 50 to 70 seconds. Heparin infusion is typically continued for 48 hours

- IV Morphine as needed for persistent chest pain or severe anxiety related to ischemia

- Check electrolytes, Keep K > 4 and Mg > 2

- Start on high intensity statin therapy such as Atorvastatin 80 mg daily and check lipid panel

- Consider beta blockers such as metoprolol 12.5 mg BID in all patients except those with hypotension, bradycardia, or heart failure

- Order ECHO and consult Cardiology

- For patients managed conservatively with noninvasive approach (No left heart catheterization), stress test can be done prior to discharge.

Orthostatic Hypotension

- Start on IV hydration, NS @ 75-100 mL/hr

- Discontinue any offending medications like diuretics and sedatives

- Continuous telemonitoring

- PT/OT consults, orthostatic vitals

Lifestyle modifications/ Nonpharmacological measures:
- Raise the head end of the bed by 20 degrees or so
- Arise slowly in stages, from supine to seated position first and then to standing
- Liberalize salt and fluid intake
- Avoiding alcohol and large meals
- Fitted compression stockings, abdominal binders

Medication trials:
- Midodrine start with 2.5 mg TID, can increase up to 10 mg TID

- Fludrocortisone 0.1 mg OD, can increase 0.1 every week (max effective dose 0.5 mg)

- Treatment of orthostatic hypotension may exacerbate supine hypertension. One strategy suggested is to treat supine hypertension at night with a transdermal nitroglycerin patch (0.025 to 0.1 mg/hour), and remove the patch in the morning prior to getting out of the bed.

Pancreatitis

- Check serum amylase, lipase, LFT's, lipid panel, and alcohol level.

- Keep NPO and start on aggressive IV hydration (NS@150 mL/hr)
- Strict input and output monitoring

- Monitor serum electrolytes (ionized Ca /Mg), supplement as indicated.

- Supportive care with pain control (Morphine, Fentanyl) and antiemetics as needed

- Ultrasound of abdomen to rule out gallstones, CBD dilation

- Start on trial of clears when appropriate, usually in 24 to 48 hours and advance to low fat diet as tolerated.

- If no significant improvement in 72 hrs or any signs of worsening, get CT abdomen with contrast.

- If CT shows evidence of necrosis, consider prophylactic antibiotics such as Imipenem/Meropenem 1 g every 8 hours **OR** Levofloxacin 750 mg IV once daily plus Metronidazole 500 mg IV every 8 hours

- If clinical condition continues to deteriorate consult Surgery for debridement of pancreatic necrosis.

- If patient is unable to tolerate orals for 4 to 5 days since admit, consult IR or GI for placement of a jejunal feeding tube to start enteral feedings. If patient cannot tolerate enteral feedings start on parenteral nutrition (TPN)

Gallstone pancreatitis:

- If biliary dilation is present without cholangitis or choledocholithiasis, get MRCP

- If signs of acute cholangitis (fever/chills or leukocytosis; with bilirubin ≥ 2 or abnormal LFT's; and biliary dilation/stone on imaging) are present, start on IV antibiotics (Zosyn **OR** Ceftriaxone **OR** Levofloxacin) and consult GI for urgent ERCP

- Cholecystectomy during same admission is recommended in patients with gallstones or biliary sludge

Pericarditis

- Suspected in patients with sharp pleuritic chest pain that tends to improve with sitting up and leaning forward

- Order EKG and CXR. EKG might show diffuse concave up ST elevations or diffuse T wave inversions. CXR look for enlarged cardiac silhouette.

- Check CBC, CMP, Troponin, ESR and CRP levels

- Start on combination therapy with NSAIDs plus Colchicine.

- NSAIDs commonly used are Ibuprofen 600 mg TID or Aspirin 650 mg TID. Once symptoms are resolved taper NSAIDs gradually over 4 to 6 weeks period.

- Colchicine 0.6 mg BID (Pt weight ≥70 kg) or 0.6 mg OD (Pt weight <70 kg) should be continued for 3 months without taper.

- In patients with contraindications to NSAIDs use glucocorticoids. Prednisone 0.2 to 0.5 mg/kg/day gradually tapered over 2 to 3 months

- Get ECHO to check LVEF and possible pericardial effusion

- Consult cardiology if trop's elevated or ECHO shows pericardial effusion or reduced LVEF

- Limit strenuous physical activity

Pneumonia

- Supplemental O2 as needed to maintain SpO2 > 92%
- ABG PRN if significant hypoxia or lethargy

- Lactic acid, PCT level, and sputum culture
- Check urine Streptococcal and Legionella antigens
- Respiratory viral panel during the fall and winter season

- Collect two sets of blood cultures and start on IV antibiotics per pneumonia protocol regimens such as
    - Ceftriaxone 1 g IV daily **plus** Azithromycin 500 mg IV or PO daily.
    - Levofloxacin 750 mg IV daily

- Patients who remain afebrile with clinical improvement can be transitioned to PO antibiotics after 48 hours. Total duration of antibiotic therapy is typically 5 to 7 days.

- Azithromycin can be discontinued after a total dose of 1500 mg. Can use Doxycycline 100 mg BID instead of Azithromycin if concern for QT prolongation.

- Patients who received Ceftriaxone as initial IV antibiotic therapy can be transitioned to Cefpodoxime (Vantin)

- Aspiration pneumonia, antibiotic options include
    - Zosyn or Unasyn (1.5 to 3 g IV every 6 hours)
    - Augmentin (875 mg PO BID)
    - Clindamycin (450 mg TID), if allergic to penicillins

- For patients with severe pneumonia and risk factors for *Pseudomonas* (COPD, chronic steroid use, gram negative bacilli in sputum) suggested empiric regimen includes combination therapy with Zosyn (4.5 g every 6 hours) or Cefepime (2 g every 8 hours) **plus** Levofloxacin (750 mg daily).

- For patients with severe pneumonia and risk factors for MRSA (ESRD, IV drug abuse, homelessness, history of MRSA, gram positive cocci in clusters in sputum) suggested empiric regimen includes combination therapy with Vancomycin (dosing per pharmacy protocol) **plus** Cefepime (2 g every 8 hours)

Hospital acquired pneumonia (HAP)

- Defined as pneumonia that occurs 48 hours or more after admission and did not appear to be incubating at the time of admission. In patients with HAP and risk factors for increased mortality or resistant organisms suggested empiric regimen includes combination therapy with Vancomycin, Cefepime and Levofloxacin.

Pulmonary Embolism (PE)

- Supplemental oxygen as needed, ABG if significant hypoxia

- D Dimer, CT angio chest
- V/Q scan (If unable to get CT angio due to renal failure or contrast allergy)

- Start on IV UFH (Unfractionated Heparin) or SubQ LMWH (Lovenox)

- Typical dosing for UFH is 80 units/kg bolus (maximum dose: 10,000 units), then 18 units/kg/hour (maximum initial infusion: 2,000 units/hour). Dosing adjustment/ monitoring should be guided per pharmacy protocol/ local hospital heparin dosing nomogram

- Typical dosing for LMWH is 1 mg/kg every 12 hours or 1.5 mg/kg once daily. Avoid use or adjust dose to 1 mg/kg once daily in patients with CrCl <30 mL/minute

- Patients with high clinical suspicion and low bleeding risk can be started on therapeutic dose anticoagulation empirically even before CT angio chest or V/Q scan is completed.

- Check EKG and start on continuous telemonitoring
- ECHO to check RVSP

- Venous duplex of bilateral lower extremities to rule out DVT

- Start on oral anticoagulation (OAC), usually after 24 hrs

Hemodynamically unstable patients

- Systemic thrombolytic therapy (tPA) or Catheter directed thrombolysis (CDT) in consultation with pulmonology and interventional radiology is recommended

- EKOS (Ultrasound assisted catheter directed thrombolysis): Ultrasonic waves are used to accelerate clot dissolution with tPA

Transitioning from IV/SubQ to oral anticoagulation:

- Warfarin: Overlap IV Heparin or SubQ Lovenox with Warfarin until INR is therapeutic x 2

- Eliquis/Xarelto: Start direct-acting oral anticoagulant (DOAC) when heparin infusion is stopped or within 2 hours prior to the next scheduled dose of Lovenox

Duration of therapy

- Provoked DVT/PE: Minimum 3 months
- First unprovoked DVT/PE: 3 months (if significant bleeding risk or patient refuses lifelong anticoagulation) to indefinite treatment (if low bleeding risk and patient agrees
- First DVT/PE with active cancer: Indefinite treatment
- Second unprovoked DVT/PE: Indefinite treatment

Pyelonephritis

- Clinical diagnosis: Cystitis symptoms (dysuria, urinary frequency/ urgency, suprapubic pain, hematuria) plus fever, chills, rigors, nausea/vomiting, flank pain or costovertebral angle tenderness

- Start on IV fluids, NS @ 100 to 125 mL/hr, monitor I/O's

- Send urine for culture/ sensitivity and blood cultures before starting antibiotics
- Start on IV antibiotics
- Antibiotic choice:
    - Ceftriaxone 1 to 2 g IV daily **or**
    - Zosyn 3.375 g IV every 6 hours **or**
    - Ciprofloxacin 400 mg IV every 12 hours

- In septic patients, get urgent CT abdomen/pelvis preferably with contrast to rule out obstruction, abscess

- In critically ill patients, start with broader spectrum antibiotics with MRSA and ESBL coverage (Vancomycin plus Meropenem)

- Indwelling catheters should be removed or replaced when possible

- Antibiotics can be switched to PO once patients are afebrile based on culture sensitivity results typically within 48 to 72 hrs

- Duration of treatment: 7 to 10 days depending on clinical course, except in patients with bacteremia who should ideally be treated for total 14 days.

QTc Prolongation/ Acquired long QT syndrome (LQTS)

- Most patients are asymptomatic. Some patients might experience palpitations, lightheadedness, or syncope.

- Increased risk of polymorphic ventricular tachycardia (Torsades de pointes) with QTc >500 milliseconds
- Start on continuous tele monitoring

- Discontinue any medications known to cause QT prolongation (such as Azithromycin, Levofloxacin, Ondansetron, Haloperidol etc.)

- Check electrolytes to exclude hypokalemia and hypomagnesemia. Keep K > 4, Mg > 2

- Magnesium sulfate 2 g IV can be given in patients even with normal magnesium level

Rhabdomyolysis

- Start on aggressive IV hydration: NS bolus 1 L, followed by NS @ 150 to 250 mL/hr

- Monitor I/O, watch for fluid overload

- Monitor CPK levels daily

- Check Urine dipstick and UA.
- Myoglobinuria if present will show positive result for blood on dipstick but without significant RBC's on microscopic urinalysis.

- Monitor for complications: renal failure, hyperkalemia, hypocalcemia, hyperphosphatemia, and hyperuricemia

- Daily CBC, CMP, Phos, Uric acid

Seizure

- Initiate seizure precautions
- Ativan PRN for seizure activity

- Get EKG and start on continuous telemonitoring
- Supplement O2 as needed, ABG if significant hypoxia
- Frequent neuro checks

- Check CBG, if hypoglycemic give thiamine 100 mg IV and 50 mL of 50% dextrose solution

- Check CPK, Lactic acid, electrolytes including magnesium, calcium levels

- Start on gentle IV hydration
- Send urine toxicology screen

- CT/ MRI and EEG in all patients with first seizure

- Neurology consult for antiseizure drug therapy in patients with second unprovoked seizure. IV Levetiracetam (Keppra) is commonly used in inpatient setting

Status epilepticus

- Defined as seizures lasting longer than 5 to 10 minutes or recurrent seizures with no return to baseline consciousness in between seizures.
- Give loading dose of Lorazepam 0.1 mg/kg IV, infused at a maximum rate of 2 mg/min, can repeat dose in 3 to 5 minutes.
- Also load with Levetiracetam (40 to 60 mg/kg, maximum 4500 mg)
- Urgent Neurology consult and continuous EEG monitoring.
- Patients who are actively seizing despite two initial doses of Lorazepam, intubate and start on continuous Midazolam or Propofol infusion

Sepsis

- Supplemental O2 as needed to maintain SpO2 >90%

- CBC, BMP, Lactic acid, PCT, ABG, CXR, UA
- Influenza screen/ viral panel during the fall and winter seasons

- Aggressive IV hydration (30mL/kg) in the form of fluid boluses completed within three hours

- Strict input/out and continuous telemonitoring
- Target MAP > 65 mmHg and urine output ≥0.5 mL/kg/hour

- Collect two sets of blood cultures before initiating antibiotics

- Start on empiric IV antibiotics such as Vancomycin (15 to 20 mg/kg IV every 8 to 12 hours as per pharmacy protocol) **plus** Zosyn (4.5 g IV every 6 hours) or Cefepime (2 g IV every 8 hours), as soon as possible.

- Repeat serum lactic acid every 2 to 4 hours, until it starts trending down

- Consider CT chest/ abdomen/pelvis if UA/CXR negative

- If patient remains hypotensive despite receiving 3 to 4 liters of fluids, start on Norepinephrine (begin 5 mcg/min, titrate to maintain MAP>65) and consult ICU

- Check cortisol, and if low with refractory hypotension consider starting on stress dose IV steroids such as Hydrocortisone 50 to 100 mg every 6 to 8 hours

- Once hemodynamically stable, antibiotics should be modified depending on suspected source of infection

- Stress ulcer prophylaxis with Pantoprazole 40 mg IV or PO daily is recommended while on stress dose steroids.

Sickle Cell Crisis (Acute Pain Episodes)

- Start on tele-monitoring and continuous pulse oximetry

- Give Morphine 4 to 10 mg IV or Dilaudid 1 to 2 mg IV every 15 minutes for 3 doses and then continue on Morphine 4 mg IV or Dilaudid 1 mg IV every 2 hours
- If no improvement in pain, consider starting on Morphine PCA (patient-controlled analgesia)

- Encourage oral fluid intake, give 1 L bolus of NS and continue on D5 1/2NS @ 100 to 150 mL/hr
- Watch for fluid overload, monitor I/O's

- Continue on home dose Hydroxyurea except in patients with severe cytopenia's and acute renal failure. If patient is not on Hydroxyurea, refer to PCP or Hem/Onc to begin Hydroxyurea as outpatient.

- Start on Oxycodone 5 to 10 mg PO every 4 to 6 hours as needed once pain is well controlled and wean off IV pain medications.

- Remember to start on DVT prophylaxis as patients tend to have a hypercoagulable state at baseline

- Daily CBC and BMP

- Avoid constipation (Senna and Colace)
- Bedside incentive spirometer

- Folic acid 1 mg PO daily

Acute chest syndrome:

- New consolidation on chest radiograph with fever or chest pain or respiratory symptoms (cough, dyspnea, wheezing, rales, hypoxia)
- Supportive care: Pain control, Hydration, Supplemental oxygen, Incentive spirometer, DVT prophylaxis)
- Transfusion: Blood transfusion, target Hb < 10 g/dL
- **Antibiotics: Cefotaxime 2 g IV every 8 hours plus Azithromycin 500 mg IV daily for total 7 days**
- Hem/onc consult

Small Bowel Obstruction (SBO)

- Bowel rest: NPO, IV fluids
- NG tube decompression if recurrent vomiting, significant abdominal distension

- BMP to check renal function and potassium levels (Supplement as needed)

- CT abdomen/pelvis with contrast (PO and IV. Avoid IV contrast if renal failure present)

- Surgical consult if CT shows complete obstruction or findings suggesting nonadhesive SBO

- Patients with adhesive SBO (previous history of abdominal surgery with no discernable causes of SBO on CT), consider Gastrografin challenge in consultation with surgery team and get follow up KUB abdominal X-ray in 12-24 hrs.

- If KUB shows contrast in colon, can start on clear liquids, and advance diet as tolerated.

- If no contrast in colon, continue conservative management in collaboration with surgery team

- Surgery is indicated if patient is deteriorating clinically or SBO lasts more than 5 days.

Stroke/ Acute Cerebrovascular Accident (CVA)

- CT head without contrast, proceed with MRI if CT negative

- Neurology consult in ED to evaluate for tPA

- Bedside swallow screen- If fails, Keep NPO until speech therapist evaluation

- Start on Aspirin 81 mg daily and high intensity statin therapy such as Atorvastatin 80 mg daily. If unable to take PO can administer Aspirin rectally

- In patients with minor ischemic stroke (NIHSS score ≤5), consider using dual antiplatelet therapy (DAPT) for 21 days. Aspirin 81 mg daily plus Plavix 75 mg daily rather than Aspirin alone.

- Patients who have a stroke while on aspirin should be considered for switching to Plavix 75 mg daily or Aggrenox (Dipyridamole extended release 200 mg/Aspirin 25 mg) after discussion with Neurology

- Check ECG and start on continuous telemonitoring

- Frequent neuro checks

- Order Carotid duplex, ECHO with bubble study

- Treat blood pressure only if SBP>220 or DBP>120 with PRN antihypertensives. No scheduled antihypertensive meds for first 48-72 hrs since admission.

- PT/OT/ST evaluations

- Check Lipid panel

Patients with AFIB

- Transient ischemic attack (TIA)
    - Can start oral anticoagulation immediately
- Small to moderate infarct
    - Repeat CT head at 48 hrs, if no hemorrhagic transformation and blood pressure controlled, can start oral anticoagulation
- Large infract
    - Wait for atleast 2 weeks before starting oral anticoagulation

Patients eligible for thrombolytic therapy

- Should receive intravenous alteplase within 4.5 hours of symptom onset

- Maintain Blood pressure at or below 180/105 mmHg during the next 24-48 hrs hours

- Anticoagulant and antithrombotic agents (such as heparin, warfarin or antiplatelet drugs) can be resumed 24 hours after the tPA infusion is completed. Follow up noncontrast CT (or MRI) scan should be obtained 24 hours after tPA is initiated before starting treatment with antiplatelet or anticoagulant agents

- Placement of Foley catheters and nasogastric tubes should be avoided for at least 24 hours

Supraventricular Tachycardia (SVT)

- Most common types of SVT are the AVNRT (atrioventricular nodal reentrant tachycardia), AVRT (atrioventricular reentrant tachycardia), and AT (atrial tachycardia)

- Hemodynamically unstable:
    - Adenosine: 6 mg rapid IV push. If no response in 1 minute, repeat with 12 mg rapid IV push

    - Cardioversion: If Adenosine not effective, proceed with immediate DC cardioversion (50 to 100J)

- Hemodynamically stable:
    - Valsalva maneuver: Patient is instructed to exhale forcefully against a closed glottis after taking in a normal breath (like straining during defecation)

- Adenosine: If Valsalva maneuver is not successful or patient unable to perform maneuver, give Adenosine 6 mg rapid IV push followed by NS flush. If no response in 2 minutes, can repeat with 12 mg rapid IV push.

- Metoprolol: If Adenosine not effective, give Metoprolol 5 mg IV every 5 minutes, maximum 3 doses (15 mg)

- Amiodarone: If all the above therapies fail, give Amiodarone bolus 150 mg over 10 minutes, then continue at 1 mg/minute for 6 hours, followed by 0.5 mg/minute for 18 hours

Syncope

- Start on gentle IV hydration
- Monitor I/O's and watch for fluid overload

- Check ECG and start on continuous telemonitoring

- Check CBG, CBC, BMP, LFTs, UA

- CT head without contrast

- Echocardiogram
- Carotid duplex

- Check Orthostatic vitals

- Discontinue offending agents/ medications

- PT/OT consults in elderly patients

- Treat underlying cause such as
    - Carotid endarterectomy for significant carotid artery stenosis

    - Pacemaker for significant bradyarrhythmia's

    - Aortic valve replacement for severe aortic stenosis

    - Liberalize salt and fluid intake in orthostatic hypotension

    - Reassurance for Vasovagal syncope

Tylenol Overdose

- Start on IV fluids, NS @ 125 mL/hour, monitor I/O's

- Check ECG and start on continuous telemonitoring

- Inform poison control and start on N-acetylcysteine (NAC) drip per protocol.

- Consider activated Charcoal if mental status is stable and presentation within 4 hours of ingestion

- If patient develops allergic reaction to NAC, stop the infusion immediately and discuss with poison control center.

- Avoid hepatotoxic drugs.
- Check salicylate level and INR
- Monitor LFT's especially ALT

- Monitor for any signs of acute liver injury, abdominal pain, coagulopathy, gastrointestinal bleeding.

- Monitor mental status closely to evaluate for any signs of encephalopathy. If mental status worsens, check ammonia level and CT head.

- Monitor blood pressure closely.

- Check repeat serum ALT and acetaminophen level approximately 18 hours after starting on NAC. If the serum ALT is elevated or acetaminophen is still detectable, recommendation is to continue treatment with NAC and continue monitoring ALT and acetaminophen levels every 12 hours thereafter. Treatment can be stopped when serum ALT is improving and acetaminophen becomes undetectable

CHM 109

Section II

ABG Basics

Normal values:

- pH: 7.35 to 7.45
- $PaCO_2$: 35 to 45 mmHg
- HCO_3: 22 to 26 mEq/L
- PaO2: 80 to 100 mmHg
- SaO_2: > 95%

Simplified Interpretation:

- Check pH: If pH < 7.4, primary disorder is acidosis, if pH > 7.4 primary disorder is alkalosis
- Check $PaCO_2$:
    - In patients with acidosis (pH < 7.4), if pCO2 > 40 acidosis is respiratory and if pCO2 ≤ 40 acidosis is metabolic
    - In patients with alkalosis (pH > 7.4), if pCO2 ≥ 40 alkalosis is metabolic and if pCO2 < 40 alkalosis is respiratory

Metabolic acidosis:

- Calculate predicted pCO2 = HCO3 + 15; or decimal digits of pH (eg, if pH is 7.27 then pCO2 should be approx. 27 mmHg)

- Check respiratory compensation:
    - If actual pCO2 within +/- 2 of predicted → proper respiratory compensation
    - If actual pCO2 > predicted pCO2 → concomitant respiratory acidosis
    - If actual pCO2 < predicted pCO2 → concomitant respiratory alkalosis

- Calculate anion gap = Na − (Cl + HCO3)
    - Normal anion gap: Diarrhea, RTA
    - Elevated anion gap (> ≈18): Lactic acidosis, Ketoacidosis (diabetes, alcohol, starvation), Renal failure

- Calculate corrected bicarb = Anion gap − 12 + HCO3
    - If corrected bicarb is between 23 to 30: Normal
    - If corrected bicarb > 30: concomitant metabolic alkalosis

- If corrected bicarb < 23: concomitant non anion gap metabolic acidosis

Metabolic alkalosis:

- Predicted pCO2 = multiple formulas but unreliable. Typically, 41 to 55 mmHg
- Check respiratory compensation:
    - If actual pCO2 between 41 to 55 → proper respiratory compensation
    - If actual pCO2 > predicted pCO2 → concomitant respiratory acidosis
    - If actual pCO2 < predicted pCO2 → concomitant respiratory alkalosis
- Common causes: Vomiting, Diuretics, Hypokalemia

Metabolic compensation in respiratory acidosis and alkalosis

For every 10 mmHg change in pCO2 from baseline of 40 mmHg	Change in Bicarb from baseline of 24 mEq/L	
	Acute	Chronic
↑ pCO2 (acidosis)	↑ 1 mEq/L	↑ 4 mEq/L
↓ pCO2 (alkalosis)	↓ 2 mEq/L	↓ 5 mEq/L

Supplemental Oxygen

High Flow Nasal Cannula (HFNC)

- Oxygen supply system capable of delivering heated and humidified oxygen at high flow rates up to 60 L/min and FiO2 up to 100%

- Typical initial setting: Flow rate 30 L/min and FiO2 60%

- Flow rate can be up titrated to 60 L/min as tolerated

- Oxygenation can be improved with increasing either flow rate or FiO2.

- Attempt to maximize flow rate first before increasing FiO2.

- High flow rates increase the nasopharyngeal airway pressure and provide a PEEP like effect

- Patients can be weaned off of HFNC once stable oxygenation (SpO2 > 92%) is achieved with flow rate ≤ 20 L/min and FiO_2 ≤ 50%

- Most commonly used in acute hypoxemic respiratory failure without hypercapnia

Oxygen delivery systems:

Device	Flow rate (L/min)	~ FiO_2 delivered
Nasal cannula	1 to 6	Up to 40%
Simple mask	6 to 10	40 to 60%
Nonrebreather mask	10 to 15	60 to 100%
OxyMask (special mask with small diffuser)	1.5 to 15	25 to 80%

Noninvasive Ventilation

Bilevel positive airway pressure (BPAP):

- Provides inspiratory positive airway pressure (IPAP) and expiratory positive airway pressure (EPAP)

- Typical initial settings: IPAP 10 cm H_2O, EPAP 5 cm H_2O, and FiO2 100%
- Backup respiratory rate can be set at 8 to 12 breaths/min (patients will receive these breaths if they fail to breathe spontaneously)

- Difference between the inspiratory and expiratory pressures (IPAP – EPAP) functions as the driving force that determines the tidal volume delivered

- To increase tidal volume, IPAP may be up titrated to a maximum of 20 cm H_2O (usually done in increments of 2 cm H_2O at a time)

- To improve oxygenation, EPAP may be up titrated to a maximum of 10 cm H_2O
- FiO2 should be adjusted to target SpO_2 >90 %
- Most commonly used in acute hypercapnic and acute hypoxemic respiratory failure

Continuous positive airway pressure (CPAP):

- Provides continuous constant positive airway pressure and essentially functions just like PEEP (Positive end expiratory pressure) used in mechanical ventilation
- Typical initial settings: CPAP level 5 to 8 cm H_2O and FiO2 100%
- Patients must initiate all breaths, no back up respiratory rate
- CPAP may be titrated up to 20 cm H_2O as tolerated
- FiO2 should be adjusted to target SpO_2 >90 %
- Most commonly used in sleep apnea and acute cardiogenic pulmonary edema

Automatic positive airway pressure (APAP/AutoPAP):

- Positive pressure delivered is automatically titrated by the machine based on resistance in patients breathing for each breath. Pressure fluctuates between minimum and maximum levels set on the machine
- Beneficial in some sleep apnea patients

Mechanical Ventilation

Typical initial settings for AC/VC (most frequently used mode in adult ICUs) mechanical ventilation

Tidal volume	6 mL/kg
Ventilator rate	14 breaths/min
PEEP	5 cm H2O
FiO2	100%
Inspiratory flow rate	60 L/min

General principles:

- Ventilator parameters are based on predicted or ideal body weight (IBW) not the actual weight of patient.

- Attempt to titrate down FiO2 to non-toxic levels (60 percent or below) as quickly as possible based on pulse oximetry (maintaining SpO_2 between 90 to 96%)

- PEEP and FiO2 affect oxygenation whereas VT and RR affect CO2 removal

- High PIP, low/normal Pplat suggests high resistance (impedance of flow in the tubing and airways) like in endotracheal tube obstruction or bronchospasm

- High PIP, high Pplat suggests low compliance (lung's ability to stretch and expand) like in interstitial pulmonary fibrosis, pneumonia, ARDS or pulmonary edema

Sedatives and analgesics:

- **Fentanyl:** Analgesic-sedative. Good choice for analgesia and sedation for most patients. Start at 25 mcg/hour, can uptitrate to 200 mcg/hour.

- **Propofol:** Hypnotic-sedative. Anticonvulsant but no analgesic effect. Watch for hypotension, bradycardia and monitor triglycerides. Start at 5 mcg/kg/minute, can uptitrate to 50 mcg/kg/minute (Use IBW in obese patients)

- **Dexmedetomidine (Precedex):** Sympatholytic- anxiolytic-analgesic-sedative. Does not cause deep sedation, allowing patients to be easily awakened. Watch for hypotension, bradycardia and occasional hypertension. Start at 0.2 mcg/kg/hour, can uptitrate to 1.5 mcg/kg/hour. (Use IBW in obese patients)

- **Midazolam (Versed):** Anxiolytic with rapid onset of action. Good choice for management of acute agitation. Start at 1 mg/hour, can uptitrate to 8 mg/hour

Neuromuscular blocking agents (Pancuronium, Rocuronium) are occasionally used in selected patients with persistent agitation despite being on multiple sedatives and analgesics.

Refer to author's website for detailed discussion
https://www.sulcusgyrus.com

EKG Basics

EKG graph paper

- Small square = 1 mm or 0.04 sec
- Large square = 5 mm or 0.2 sec

Normal values:

- Heart Rate: 60 to 100 beats/min
- P Wave: width < 3 small boxes (0.12 sec) and height < 2.5 small boxes (0.25 mv)
- PR Interval: 3 to 5 small boxes (0.12 to 0.20 sec)
- QRS duration: < 3 small boxes (0.12 sec)
- T wave: < 5 small boxes in limb leads, < 10 small boxes in precordial leads

Heart rate estimation:

- Regular rhythm: Division of 300 by number of large squares between consecutive R waves
- Irregular rhythm: Number of QRS complexes (R waves) on the EKG strip x 10

Rhythm analysis:

- Regular rhythm: Interval between R waves is constant or varies by < 1.5 small boxes
- Irregular rhythm: Interval between R waves varies by > 1.5 small boxes

Systematic Interpretation:

- Read EKG strip from left to right
- Seven step approach
    - Calculate heart rate
    - Check rhythm
    - Assess P Wave
        - Present or absent?
        - Occurring regularly or irregularly?
        - P wave before each QRS or not?
        - Shape
    - Measure PR interval
        - Beginning of P wave to onset of QRS complex
    - Measure QRS duration
        - Beginning of Q wave to end of S wave
    - Look at ST segment

- Elevated, depressed or isoelectric to TP segment?
  - T waves
    - Tall, inverted or biphasic?

Sinus Rhythms (Impulse originates in SA node; normal P waves, normal QRS)

- Normal sinus rhythm
- Sinus bradycardia
- Sinus tachycardia
- Sinus arrhythmia
- Sinus pause/arrest

Atrial Rhythms: (Impulse originates in atrial tissue; +/− P waves, Normal QRS)

- Atrial flutter
- Atrial fibrillation (AFib)
- Supraventricular tachycardia (SVT)
- Premature atrial complexes (PACs)
- Multifocal atrial tachycardia (MAT)

Ventricular Rhythms (Impulse originates in ventricles; no P waves, Wide QRS)

- Ventricular tachycardia (VT)
- Premature ventricular complexes (PVCs)
- Torsades de Pointes
- Ventricular fibrillation (VFib)

Refer to author's website for detailed discussion
https://www.sulcusgyrus.com

Supplement I:

Simplified clinical classification of commonly isolated pathogens

GPC's	GPR's
Staphylococcus	Commensals/Contaminants (Skin)
Streptococcus	Clostridia (Wound)
Enterococcus	Listeria (CSF)
GNC's	GNR's
Neisseria	Enterobacteriaceae
Moraxella	Pseudomonas
	Legionella
Atypical	
Mycoplasma	
Chlamydia	

Frequently used antibiotics in clinical practice with coverage spectrum

Penicillins
Unasyn (Ampicillin + Sulbactam), Augmentin (Amoxicillin + Clavulanate), Zosyn (Piperacillin + Tazobactam)
- Good coverage: MSSA, streptococci, enterococci, enteric GNR's and anaerobes

Cephalosporins
All cephalosporins have poor coverage against enterococcus and anaerobes

First generation: Ancef (Cefazolin), Keflex (Cephalexin)
- Good coverage: MSSA, streptococci

Third generation: Ceftriaxone
- Good coverage: Streptococci, enteric GNR

Fourth generation: Cefepime

- Good coverage: MSSA, Streptococci and enteric GNR's

Fluoroquinolones
Most fluoroquinolones have poor coverage against enterococcus and anaerobes

Levofloxacin
- Good coverage: Enteric GNR's, Atypicals, Streptococcus pneumoniae, Haemophilus influenzae

Ciprofloxacin
- Good coverage: Enteric GNR's, Haemophilus influenzae

Vancomycin
- Good gram positive coverage (MSSA, MRSA, Streptococci) but poor gram negative coverage.
- PO Vancomycin is effective against Clostridium difficile

Supplement II:

Options for oral treatment of Methicillin-Resistant *Staphylococcus Aureus* (MRSA)

Clindamycin 300 to 450 mg PO TID to QID
Trimethoprim-sulfamethoxazole 1 to 2 DS tablets PO BID
Doxycycline 100 mg PO BID
Linezolid 600 mg PO BID

Commonly used antipseudomonal antibiotics

- Ceftazidime 2 g IV every 8 hours
- Cefepime 2 g IV every 8 hours
- Levofloxacin 750 mg PO or IV once daily
- Meropenem 1 g IV every 8 hours
- Piperacillin-tazobactam (Zosyn) 4.5 g IV every 6 hours

Enterococcus UTI

Oral options
Nitrofurantoin 100 mg BID x 5 days
Amoxicillin 500 mg TID x 5 days
Fosfomycin 3 g single dose
Ciprofloxacin 250 mg BID x 3 days (500 mg BID x 7 days in case of complicated UTI)

Intravenous options
Ampicillin
Unasyn
Zosyn
Vancomycin

VRE - Linezolid, Daptomycin

ESBL producing organisms

- Carbapenems (such as Meropenem 1 g IV every 8 hours) are the drug of choice
- Fosfomycin 3 g PO single dose is usually effective for cystitis caused by ESBL-producing *E. coli*

Supplement III:

Peri-operative anticoagulation management

Assess thromboembolic risk:
- A Fib: High risk (CHADS2 score 5-6), Medium risk (3-4), Low risk (0-2)
- Prosthetic valve: High risk
- VTE: High risk (diagnosed < 3 months), Medium risk (3-12 months), Low risk (>12 months)

Assess bleeding risk:
- Procedure plus patient
- Any procedure lasting >45 minutes is considered High risk

Timing of interruption:
- Warfarin 5 days before procedure
- Other agents 3 days before procedure

Bridging need with IV heparin
- Depends on thromboembolic risk
    - High risk: Yes
    - Medium risk: maybe
    - Low risk: No, generally

Re-start: Safe to resume oral anticoagulants morning after uncomplicated surgery

Cosyntropin stimulation test

- Cosyntropin 250 mcg IV bolus (standard high-dose test)
- Serum cortisol is measured before, 30 and 60 minutes after giving Cosyntropin
- Normal adrenal function is indicated by serum cortisol level ≥ 18 mcg/dL before or after cosyntropin injection

Commonly used Insulins

Generic	Brand name	Onset (minutes)	Duration (hours)
Aspart	Novolog	15	3 to 5
Lispro	Humalog	15	3 to 5
Regular	Humulin R Novolin R	30	5 to 8
NPH	Humulin N Novolin N	60	12 to 16
Detemir	Levemir	60	20 to 24
Glargine	Lantus	60	20 to 24
70% NPH plus 30% Regular	Humulin 70/30 Novolin 70/30	30	12 to 16

Common causes of elevated BNP

AFIB (atrial fibrillation)
Burns
CHF (congestive heart failure)
COPD (chronic obstructive pulmonary disease)
Cirrhosis
OSA (obstructive sleep apnea)
PE (pulmonary embolism, acute)
PHT (pulmonary hypertension)
Renal failure
Stroke
Sepsis

Of Note: Cirrhosis, renal failure, stroke and sepsis are also associated with elevated D-dimer levels

Lactic acidosis

Type A lactic acidosis
- Caused by tissue hypoperfusion
- Shock, sepsis, and heart failure

Type B lactic acidosis
- Caused by toxin related impairment of cellular metabolism
- DKA, alcoholism, HIV, certain malignancies and drugs like Metformin, Linezolid

Massive transfusion

- Check PT/PTT/INR and platelet count after every 5 units of pRBC transfusion.
- If dilutional coagulopathy present (PT/PTT > 1.5 times control) give two units of FFP. If platelet count falls < 50,000 give one unit platelets.
- Monitor potassium and calcium levels

Supplement IV:

Cardiac arrest/ Code Blue

Resuscitation begins with circulation, followed by airway opening, and then rescue breathing (C-A-B).

- Confirm no pulse, start CPR immediately
- Insert oropharyngeal or nasopharyngeal airway and begin bag-valve-mask (BVM)/ Ambu bag ventilation with 100% oxygen (compression to ventilation ratio 30:2)
- Attach monitor/defibrillator and check rhythm
- Shock if VF/pVT, and resume CPR immediately for 2 mins. If monitor shows asystole/PEA give Epinephrine 1 mg IV and continue CPR for 2 mins.
- Switch chest compressor and do pulse/rhythm check every 2 mins.
- Continue giving Epinephrine every 3 to 5 mins.
- If subsequent rhythm checks reveal persistent VT/VF nonresponsive to

defibrillation, give Amiodarone 300 mg IV bolus, can repeat another dose of 150 mg.
- Endotracheal intubation can be deferred until after return of spontaneous circulation (ROSC)
- Contact family and consider termination of CPR after 20 mins if no ROSC and family agreeable otherwise continue CPR for full 40 mins. If still no ROSC CPR can be terminated.

Made in the USA
Las Vegas, NV
15 June 2024